Production Technology of *Bergenia ciliata* (Haw.) Sternb.
A golden herb of Himalaya

By
Sibdas Baskey
Bandan Thapa
Koushik Roy
Sarad Gurung

Globally cultivation of medicinal plants has made a phenomenal progress. The growth of production of this multipurpose plant also has changed dramatically in the recent past due to crop improvement and advancement in production technology. In India North Eastern Himalayan range is enriched with many valuable herbs and their superior genotype. Himalaya is known for its rich and diverse plant wealth from time immemorial. The diversity of this resource is quite pronounced both horizontally and vertically. The Darjeeling Himalaya harbors a diverse genotype of Berginia and it is used as the herbal medicinal practices by among all ethno-cultural groups of this region. It is already exploited at a large scale which is going to be threatened their existence due to over harvesting for getting quick money depending on natural population. The status of this plant in the context of their existence, exploitation and usage requires considerable attention due to its alarming depletion of population. There is huge demand of this herb in market so an immediate attention towards documentation of the status, usage and potential in this of this plant is required.

Concerted research efforts are being made by the scientists around the world to adopt, apply and evaluate the methodology for conservation of this herb and improving crop yield. Understanding and prediction of crop response to environment is the major theme which may further help to identify improved crop management practices.

This book is a mixture of theoretical and applied investigation together with a number of studies of current research programmes and innovative and successful crop cultivation strategies done in Regional Research Centre (Hill Zone), UBKV, Kalimpong along its adjoining parts like Lava, Pedong Algarah, etc. The focus is on conservation and increase in population of this endangered with certain improved management techniques. The book is the result of a

4

collective effort of scientist from various disciplines of this institution. The output made by the scientist will serve as a valuable reference for researchers, teachers and student. We will be happy if the book will ultimately serve the purpose of scientists, educational researchers, farmers and different companies engaged in research work and commercial cultivation of this valuable endangered plant in a meaningful way.

Sibdas Baskey
Bandan Thapa
Koushik Roy
Sarad Gurung

Acknowledgement

Pakhanbhed, an important golden herb of Himalaya has become a subject of great interest recently due to its immense capacity to dissolve kidney stone. First of all, fervently and modestly we express our deep sense of gratitude to Prof. (Dr.) Debashis Mojumder, Honourable Vicc-chancellor for his keen interest and moral support for the preparation of this manuscript regarding outcome of various research findings of this herb.

'We are immensely grateful to Prof. Ashok Choudhury, Director of Research, for his valuable advice and thought provoking suggestion, which greatly help us to develop a keen research aptitude regarding this valuable plant and develop this manuscript in a fruitful way.

'We express our sincerest and heart felts gratitude to Dr. Jitendra Kumar, Director, ICAR-Directorate of Medicinal and Aromatic Plants for his valuable guidance, keen and continued interest, encouragement with constructive suggestions throughout the course of research work which ultimately helped us to infer our research findings.

The support and hard work provided by the staff members of AICRP on MAP& B is highly acknowledged. Our special thanks to Forest officers (DFO) and Range officer, whose immense experience and Knowledge, we have utilized in ample measures to build up the Berginia information base. This work would have been impossible without the co-operation of the people living in the area who helped us during the field visits.

The help extended by the scientists of the Regional Research Station (Hill Zone), Kalimpong are gratefully acknowledged. We are extremely grateful to the ADR, UBKV (HZ), Kalimpong, Darjeeling for generous financial assistance for this programme.

Sibdas Baskey
Bandan Thapa
Koushik Roy
Sarad Gurung

Introduction

Bergenia ciliata (Haw.) Sternb. is rhizomatous, evergreen, perennial herb. It belongs to family Saxifragaceae. It is popularly known as Pakhanbed; pigsqueak, due to the sound produced when two leaves are rubbed together; elephant's ears , due to the shape of the leaves, and large rockfoil. This family, Saxifragaceae, comprises of 30 genera and 580 species, mostly distributed in the cold and temperate Himalayas and Central and Eastern Asia between 4000 to 12000 feet. The genus *Bergenia* comprises about 6 species distributed in temperate Himalayas and central and Eastern Asia. Hooker (1888) and Wehmer (1948) have reported three species of *Bergenia* from India. It is a good source of bergenin. It has many medicinal properties such as antibacterial, anti-inflammatory, anticancer, antidiabetic. It is used mainly for kidney disorder. Its phytochemical constituents are Gallic acid, Tannic acid, (-)-3-0- Galloylepicatechin, (-)-3-0-Galloylcatechin, (+)-Catechin, Gallicin.The demand of pakhanbhed has increased manifold in the last two decades. Now, cultivation is a viable option to get high profit as having high market demand due to decreasing production in natural forests. It is important both economically and ecologically for the farming community of Darjeeling Himalaya. It could become an effective component for rural development in the north-eastern states as its cultivation needs low input and labour and generates a very attractive economic return.

Names of *Bergenia ciliata* in different languages

Languages	Names
Sanskrit	Pashanbheda
Hindi	Pakhenbhed
Nepalese	Pakanabadha
Sinhalese	Pahanabeya
Japanese	Yukinoshita
German	Steinbrech
Unani	Mukha
Arabian	Junteyenah
Persian	Gashah
Gujrati	Pashanbheda
Assamese	Patharkuchi
Kannada	Alepgaya, Pahanbhedi, Hittaga
Kashmir	Pashanbhed
Marathi	Pashanbheda
Oriya	Pasanbhedi, Pashanabheda
Tamil	Sirupilai
Punjabi	Kachalu, Pashanbhed
Telugu	Kondapindi

Malayalam	Kallurvanchi, Kallurvanni, Kallorvanchi

Botanical Classification

Kingdom : Plantae

Subkingdom : Tracheobionta

Superdivison : Spermatophyta

Division : Magnoliphyta

Class : Magnoliopsida

Subclass : Rosidae

Order : Rosales

Family : Saxifragaceae

Genus : *Bergenia*

Species : *Ciliata*

Synonyms:

Bergenia ciliata (Haw.) Sternb.

Megasea ciliata (Haw.)

Saxifraga ciliata (Haw.) Royle.

Saxifraga ligulata Wall.

Saxifraga thysanodes Lindl

Habitat

It is found in Afghanistan, South Tibet, Bhutan (Phuntsoling district, Deothang district, Ha district and Mongar district. In India, it is found in Himalayas (Kumaon), Meghalaya, Lushai hills, West Bengal (Darjeeling, Labha, Takdah, Rimbick, Kalimpong), Arunachal Pradesh (Nyam Jang Chu), Sikkim (Kyongnosla, Changu, Karponanag, Lachen to Thongu, Nathang, Prekchu-Tsokha, Pangolakha-Subaney Dara, Gangtok) (Hafid *et al.,* 2009, Grierson, 1987, Anon, 2001)

Plant Description

These plants are clump-forming, rhizomatous, and evergreen in nature. It is a perennial herb with short, thick, fleshy and procumbent stems and very stout rootstock. Leaves are ovate or round and often have wavy or saw-toothed edges and are spirally arranged rosette of leaves 6–35 cm long and 4–15 cm broad. Leaves turn to bright red with short stiff hairs and attain about 30 cm lengths in the autumn. Upper and lower surfaces of leaves are hairy, becoming almost hairless in age. Flowering period is usually March-May. The flowers grow on a stem similar in colour to a rhubard stalk and most genotypes have cone-shaped flowers in varying shades of pink. These can range from almost white to ruby red and purple. (The Garden Helper, 2009).Flowers are usually 3.2 cm in diameter, forming a cymose panicle with flexible flowering stem, 10-25 cm long leafless and styles (Kritikar and Basu,2005, Kindersley, 2008, Anon,2002, Anon,1988).

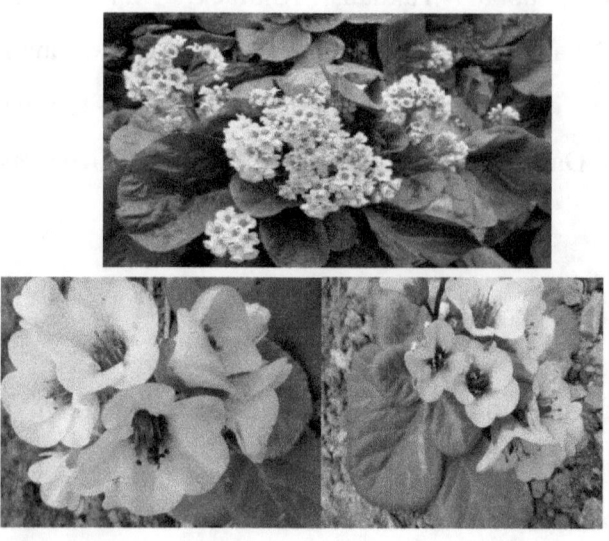

Fig 1. Flowers of different genotype of Pakhanbhed

Macroscopic features

The rhizomes are compact solid, barrel shaped, somewhat cylindrical, measuring 1-3 cm long and 1-2 cm in diameter. The outer surface is brown coloured with small roots, ridges, furrows wrinkles and covered with root scars. It possesses aromatic odor and astringent taste (Mehra *et al.,* 1971, Srivastava *et al.,* 2008).

Microscopic features

Transverse section of rhizome shows cork divided into two zones; outer and inner. Outer zone is with few layers of slightly compressed and brown coloured cells whereas inner zone is multilayered consisting of thin walled, tangentially elongated and colourless cells. Cork is followed by single layered cambium and two to three layers of secondary cortex. Cortex consists of a narrow zone of parenchymatous cells containing a number of simple starch grains whereas most of cortical cells contain large rosette crystals of calcium oxalate (CaC_2O_4) and starch grains. Endodermis and pericycle are absent whereas vascular bundles arranged on a ring. Cambium is present as continuous ring composed of two to three layers of thin walled, tangentially elongated cells. Xylem consists of fibres, tracheids, vessels and parenchyma. Centre is occupied by large pith composed of circular to oval parenchymatous cells containing starch grains with CaC_2O_4 crystals similar to those found in cortical region. Vessels with simple pits have perforation plates on one end or at both ends and tracheids have helical thickenings (Mehra *et al.*, 1971, Srivastava *et al.*, 2008, Manjunatha, 2010)

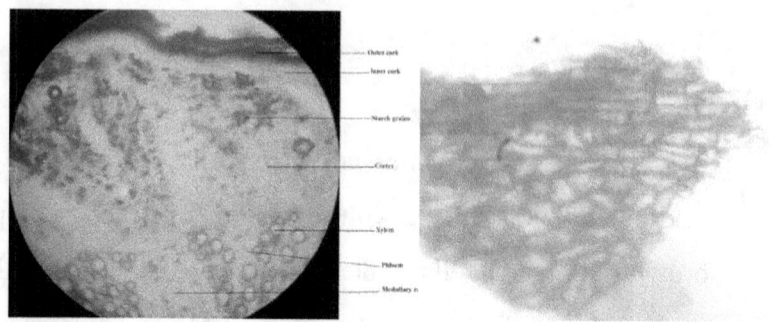

Fig. i. T.S. of *Bergenia ciliata* Rhizome   Fig. ii. Cork cells

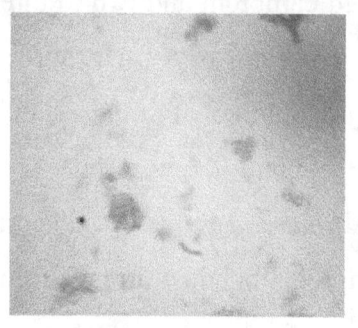   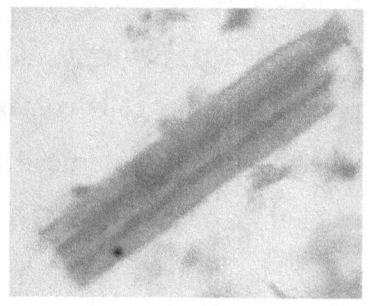

Fig. iii. Starch grains   Fig. iv. Xylem Vessels

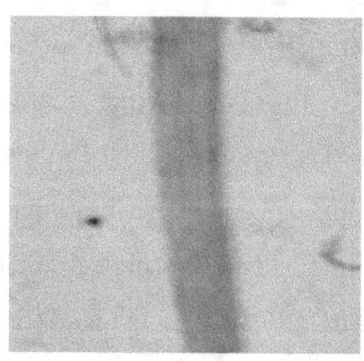   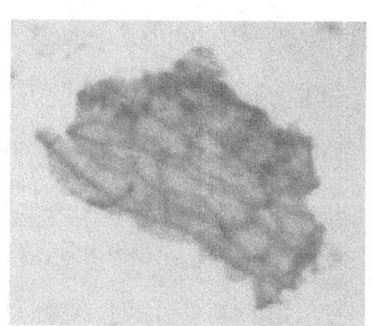

Fig. v. Fibers   Fig. vi. Parenchyma cell

Fig. 2. T.S. of different parts of *Bergenia ciliata*

14

Agro-techniques for *Berginia ciliata*

Climate requirements

It is cultivated as rain fed crop in Sikkim, Arunachal Pradesh, Darjeeling (West Bengal), Assam and Meghalaya. It tolerates the temperatures ranging from 10-37 ^{0}C. The plant requires a hot moist climate and an elevation between 100 and 2100 m for its cultivation. It can be grown successfully even in areas which receive heavy rainfall with high relative humidity.

Soil requirement

It can be cultivated successfully in organic matter rich fertile, well drained forest soils. Soils with high organic matter content and moisture holding capacity are also suitable for cultivation. However, light, porous and well-drained soil rich in organic content is most suitable for its cultivation. The leaf colour is best when plants are grown in a poor soil in a sunny position. It is not grown well in cold winds. The plant is hardy. The flowers and young leaves are sensitive to frost, so it is best to choose a position with shade from the early morning sun. This species is only hardy in sheltered gardens of Darjeeling Himalaya. If the leaves are cut back by frost then they are soon replaced by fresh leaves in the spring. It can be successfully cultivated in full sun or light shade in most soils, but prefers a deep fertile soil that does not dry out fully. It grows well in heavy clay soils. Plants are at their best in a medium-heavy soil. It can stand in wide range of soil, pH ranging acid, neutral and basic (alkaline). It can grow in semi-shade (light woodland) or no shade. It prefers moist soil.

Propagation

Propagation can be achieved by both seed and rhizome. Seeds should be sown in surface soil in a greenhouse or 70% agro-shade-net house for preparing mother nursery. The soil of the nursery should be well composed, rich in organic matter and moisture content should be normal, it should not be dry out. Seed germination rate is not enough in normal condition and it usually takes 1-6 months for seed germination at 15^0C (Rice, 1988). Seed viability can also be lost in very short period of time. It is better, Fresh seeds should be sown for raising seedling. Fresh seeds germinate better than stored seeds. It needs seed priming for getting expectable germination rate. Two weeks cold stratification at 4^0C can speed up germination. When Seedling are larger enough to handle, prick the seedlings out and transferred them into pot-trays and grow them on in light shade in the greenhouse for at least their first winter. Then transplanting can be done into main field in late spring or early summer. Smaller rhizome of about 2-3 cm thickness can be planted at spacing of 10X10 cm in nursery. The rate of growth is slow and as it takes about 18 months time for raising plants in nursery for field planting.

Nursery Technique

It takes about one month to develop a mother nursery which can supply planting material for raising cultivation.

Propagation through Rhizome

The crop can be raised by direct planting of 7.5-12.5 cm long rhizome segments (average weight: 23-26 gm) with 2-3 nodes as propagation material for quick and faster regeneration in the field in late summer or onset of monsoon. It is treated with 100 ppm IBA solution for two minutes. Raising crop through rhizome segments can reduce crop cycle by one year in comparison to propagation through seed sown. However, it requires large quantity of rhizome sections for planting. It is noted that the smaller rhizome segments of about 2 cm thickness can be planted at spacing of 10X10 cm in nursery. The rate of growth is slow and as it takes about 18 months time for raising plants in nursery for field planting.

Propagation by Seed

The seeds are very minute in shape and exhibit poor viability and germination potential. They exhibit slightly recalcitrant nature and need to be used immediately after maturity in spring season (March-April). The seed is stratified for 15 days at 4°C to improve germination. Storing will lose viability. Seeds are sown over top surface of raised beds or poly bags over the moist layer of forest litter or farmyard manure preferably under greenhouse conditions. The seeds take 60-90 days for germination. After germination, the seedlings are picked out at two-three leave stage and planted in fresh nursery beds at spacing of 10X10 cm and takes a season to grow large before planting in the field in next summer.

Rate of Planting material

88,000-90,000 plants are usually required needed to plant one hectare land.

Land Preparation

Land preparation should be done before or during March and debris are either burnt or removed from the field. Raised bed should generally be prepared 15-20 cm from ground level and the soil must be fine and have optimum moisture. The length of the bed may be kept 2 to 3 meter and width is restricted to a maximum of 1 meter only to facilitate intercultural operations. The farmyard manure and leaf manure at equal proportion are mixed in each bed soil before planting. The spacing may vary with the type of land being used for cultivation. However, good yield can be obtained when it is cultivated on fertile lands.

Fertilization

Nutrient management is a key component for good growth and development of this plant. This prefers to grow where friable soil with rich in humus content. Usually, farmer should not apply any nutrient in their field at high altitude range because most of the hilly soils are rich in humas and high organic matter. However, at lower elevation (800-1300 m asl) farmer apply roughly FYM and leaf manure.

Our study at Kalimpong (1250 m asl) revealed that vermicompost is very important as because of mixture of worm casts enriched with macro and micronutrients (N, P, K, Mn., Fe, Mo, B, Cu and Zn.), The nutrient level of vermicompost (1-1.5% N, 0.6-0.8% P and 1.2-1.5 K) is higher than any other compost (Table 2). However, farmer can go for other farm household refused to enrich their soil fertility for healthy growth of the plant.

Application of manure

It can be grown without chemical fertilizers and use of organic pesticides, organic manures like farm yard manure (FYM), vermi-compost and green manure etc. may be used as per the need (Table 1). Split application of decomposed manure is preferable. Apply first dose of manue (2/3) before the sowing of transplanted plant.

Table 1: Organic inputs recommendation on observation basis at field level.

Input	Quantity required (t/ha)	Remarks
Neem / Pongamiacake	0.50	Protection against termite and other soil borne pest and pathogen.
FYM	10.00	There is possibility of weed infestation and poor establishment of the crop.
Compost	10.00	Possibility of weed and pathogen infestation and poor establishment of the crop.
Vermicompost	0.50	This source is totally weed free and help in better performance of the crop.

Table 2: Average nutrient content of bulky manure which may apply to Berginia

Manure	Percent Content		
	N_2	P_2O_5	K_2O
1. Animal Refuse			
Cattle dung, fresh	0.3-0.4	0.1-0.2	0.1-0.3
Night soil, fresh	1.0-1.6	0.8-1.2	0.2-0.6
Poultry manure, fresh	1.0-1.8	1.4-1.8	0.8-0.9
2. Wood Ashes			
Ash, household	0.5-1.9	1.6-4.2	2.3-12.0
Ash, wood	0.1-0.2	0.8-5.9	1.5-36.0
3. Farm Factory and Habitation			
Rural compost, dry	0.5-1.0	0.4-0.8	0.8-1.2
Urban compost, dry	0.7-2.0	0.9-3.0	1.0-2.0

FYM, dry	0.4-1.5	0.3-0.9	0.3-1.9
4. Plant Residues			
Rice hulls	0.3-3.5	0.2-0.5	0.3-0.5
Straw and stalks: Banana, dry	0.61	0.12	1.0
Maize	0.42	1.57	1.65
Paddy	0.36	0.08	0.71
Wheat	0.53	0.10	1.10

Planting Time

It is a hardy plant. Hence, it can be planted in spring as well as summer in the hills. The best time for planting is monsoon time (June -July).

Transplanting

Land preparation should be completed before or during March. It is generally planted at the onset of monsoon during May - June, when soil has sufficient moisture for plant establishment.FYM can be applied during the land preparation to get better yield. The rooted plants or the seedling can be transplanted in the field maintaining proper spacing.

Spacing

Plant to plant distance should be 30X30 cm in main field in 12-15 cm raised bed gives better yields.

Intercropping System

The maximum height of plants which can be achieved under optimum growing conditions may be 30 cm with heavy leaf biomass.

Intercropping can be possible with comparatively short duration crop Kalmegh (*Andrographis paniculata*) with erect type growth habits

Intercultural operation

It is water lodge sensitive crop. Water stagnation should be avoided. The leaves of plants are prone to decay during rainy season. Decaying leaves must be removed immediately from the plants to avoid any fungal infection. Weeds and grasses are common during rainy season which should be uprooted immediately. As and when required, weeding should be done to keep the field clean. Generally, one times weeding operation should be done per month.

Irrigation Practices

Requirement of irrigation depends upon the climatic conditions. For seed germination field should be irrigated with light sprinkler shower one-two day's interval. Heavy irrigation will misplace the seed and some time due to anaerobic condition for long period leads to poor germination. In main field, it need not required any fixed irrigation, however, intermittent application two in fortnight is require. Sprinkler irrigation can be tried to keep the humidity level high at canopy level. It can tolerate dryness, but its growth gets affected when the moisture goes down the optimal level (i.e. field capacity) for the plant. It may be watered intermittently 15 day's interval during November to April. The nursery beds and fields after plantation should be irrigated periodically as and when required weekly or fortnightly. Regular irrigation during lean period may be given a must for proper growth and flowering of plant.

Pest management

Clean cultivation should be followed. Leaf hopper and snails attack the foliar part of crop. No bacterial and fungal diseases were reported yet. To check the disease, the extra foliar growth and decaying leaf should be removed. Sometimes extreme frost conditions are observed in high hills which lead to leaf and flower decay.

Harvesting

The crops mature from the second year and onwards. However, it is better to harvest roots during third year.

Post-harvest Management

Proper drying of harvested material is essential to ensure quality. The underground rhizomes are taken out. After removing the leaf and soil debris, rhizomes are washed thoroughly under running water and cut it into small pieces of 5 cm long and allowed to dry in partial shade for 8-10days or till complete drying (4-6% moisture stage). The dry rhizomes are packed in gunny bags and stored in cool and dry conditions. The rhizome usually contains bergenin (0.6%), gallic acid and tannic acid (14.2%), glucose (5.6%, mucilage and wax).

Yield

The plant yields 7.0-7.2 tonnes rhizomes per hectare (dry biomass) after second year when the crop is raised through rhizome cuttings.

Cost of Cultivation

Cost of production may vary from different agro-climatic situation. However, The cost of cultivation for one hectare may come to Rs.75,000/-.

Calendar of operation

CALENDER OF OPERATION FOR NURSERY	
March-April	Selection of site for nursery, cleaning the site.
May-June	Filling the pit/trench with top soil, FYM, Compost and planting of rhizome and mulching sowing of seeds.
July	Planting of rhizomes may be continued.
August	Monitoring the nurseries.
September-October	Weeding and application of organic manures.
November-December	Erection of shades in high altitudes suckers from low temperature and frost.
January-Febuary	Mulching and irrigation.

Month	Activities (crop calendar for Main field)
December-January	Provide shade in nurseries at higher altitude to reduce damage due to frost.
Febuary-March	Filling the pit/trench with top soil, FYM, Compost and planting of rhizome and mulching.
April-May	Monitor the plantation.
June –July	New rhizomes can be planted from nursery to main fields.
August	Monitor the plantation.
September-October	Harvesting in the low and mid altitude. Follow the phytosanitary measures.
November-December	Harvesting in the high altitude. Follow the Phytosanitary measures.

Historical review (Ayurvedic) of Pashanbheda

Different Ayurvedic treatise mentioned this plant and recommended its uses for treatment of urinary stones. Charak Samhita (210 BC-170 AD) mentioned this plant under the name Pashanbhed and recommended it for painful micturition, for curing abdominal tumour and for breaking up calculi. Sushruta Samhita (170 BC-340BC) and Ashtang Hridaya (341 AD-434AD) also do mention it for uric acid calculi.

Ayurvedic uses

Pashanbheda is used in Ayurveda and Unani system of medicine for treatment of many diseases especially for urinary stones. It is *shita* in *virya*, bitter in taste and has *bhedana* and *basti-shodhana* actions. It is indicated in the stone, *mutra-kricchra* and *shula* (Bhavaprakasha

Haritakyadi Varga:184-185) The plant roots has cooling, laxative, analgesic, abortifacient (abortion causing) and aphrodisiac properties.

The roots are used in treatment of vesicular calculi, urinary discharges, excessive uterine haemorrhage, diseases of the bladder, dysentery, mennorrhagia, splenic enlargement and heart diseases. Ayurveda mentions, the roots as bitter, acrid, post digestion pungent and cool in potency. It is tridoshnashak (balances Vata, Pitta and Kapha).

- Teething troubles: The roots are rubbed down and given with honey to children when teething.
- Ear pain: The leave juice is extracted in mortar and pestle. This is used as ear drops to cure earache.
- Intestinal parasite roundworms: About 10gm of root paster or juice is taken orally by human adults with molasses, twice a day for 3-4 days.
- Cuts,boils,wounds and burns: Dried roots paste is applied externally on affected body parts.
- Urinary disorder,stomach disorders and urogential complaints: Decoction of fresh roots is taken orally for treating these conditions.
- Constipation: Root paste is taken with lukewarm water.
- Dysentry: Approximately 5-10gm root powder is taken with fresh water two times a day.
- Fever: The root powder tea is given to treat fever.
- Cough: 50ml root decoction with candy sugar is given for one week.

IDENTITY, PURITY AND STRENGTH
(a) **Foreign matter:** Not more than 2 per cent.
(b) **Total Ash:** Not more than 13 per cent.

(c) **Acid-insoluble ash**: Not more than 0.5 per cent.

(d) **Alcohol-soluble extractive:** Not less than 9 per cent.

(e) **Water-soluble extractive: Not** less than 15 per cent.

PROPERTIES AND ACTION

(i) Rasa : Tikta, Kasaya

(ii) Guna : Laghu

(iii) Virya : sita

(iv) Vipaka : Katu

(v) Karma : Bhedana, Vastisodhana, Asmarighna, Mutravirecaniya

IMPORTANT FORMULATIONS - Asmarihara Kasaya Curna, Mutravirecaniya Kasaya Curna

THERAPEUTIC USES - Asmari, Meha, Mutrakicchra

DOSE – It can be taken 3-6 g of the drug in powder form or 20-30 g of the drug for decoction.

Traditional Knowledge of Pashanbhed used by local people of India

Ailments	Plant Parts Used	Method Used	Community Reported Used
Kidney and Gall bladder stone	Rhizome	Dried powder is used	Local knowledgeable person, Van Rawat, Bhotiya and Illiterate local people.
Wound / old wounds	Leaves and Rhizomes	Powder of dried leaves and rhizome are applied to heal old	Local illiterate people, Buxa and Van Rawat

26

		wounds	
Septic	Rhizome	Paste of rhizome used as antiseptic	Locals and Van Rawat
Cough and cold	Leaves and Rhizome	Leaves and rhizome boiled with water and given in cold and cough.	Bhotiya
Cut and Burns	Rhizome	Crushed rhizome mixed with curd and applied on burns	Bhotiya and Van Rawat
Dysentery and Diarrhoea	Rhizome	Infusion of rhizome is taken orally for diarrhoea and dysentery	Locals, Van Rawat and Bhotiya
Fever	Rhizome	Dried powder is given in fever	Buxa
Asthama	Rhizome	Rhizome juice is given in acute asthama	Van Rawat and Buxa
Gasto-intestinal problems	Rhizome	All kinds of intestinal problems are cured by chewing fresh rhizome	Local literate and illiterate people
Eye ailments	Rhizome	Crushed rhizome sap is applied in eye diseases	Local knowledgeable people, Van Rawat and Bhotiya
Septic pimples developed on the head of new born baby (Laizi)	Rhizome	Rhizome paste is applied	Local people, Bhotiya and Van Rawat
Chronic ulcers	Rhizome	The rhizome is crushed and used in all	Van Rawat and Bhotiya

		kinds of ulcers	
Cutaneous infections	Rhizome	Rhizome paste is effective in cutaneous diseases	Local people
Inflammation	Rhizome	Paste of fresh rhizome is used	Local people
Rheumatic	Rhizome	Rhizome paste is anti rheumatic	Local people
Helmintic	Rhizome	Fresh & dried rhizome extract is used orally	Bhotiya
Piles	Rhizome	Fresh & dried rhizome extract is used orally	Buxa, Bhotiya and Local people
Tonsils	Leaves and Rhizome	Rhizome & leaves paste is applied externally	Bhotiya and Van Rawat
Cardiac problems	Rhizome	Rhizome powder is given	Bhotiya
Colitis	Rhizome	Rhizome paste cure internal wounds including colitis	Bhotiya
Aphrodisiac	Rhizome	Rhizome powder is given to increase spermatozoa	Bhotiya
Urinary diseases	Rhizome	Rhizome sap is taken orally in all kind of urinary problems	Locals, Van Rawat, Bhotiya and Buxa

Phytochemistry

It consists of major phenolic compound 'bergenin' (nearly 0.9 %) and other phenolic compounds in minor amount (Udupa *et al.,*1970, Jain and Gupta,1962, Roy and Philip,1981,Umashankar *et al.,*1997).Phenolic compounds includes (+)- afzelechin (Tucci *et al.,* 1969),leucocyanidin, gallic acid, tannic acid, methyl gallate (Dixit *et. al.,*1989), (+)-catechin, (+)-catechin -7-O-ß-D-glucopyranoside, 11-O-galloyl bergenin (Umashankar *et al.,*1997); a lactone-Paashaanolactone (Chandrareddy *et al.,*1998)It also contains sterols *viz.,* sitoindoside I, ß- sitosterol and ß-sitosterol-D-glucoside, glucose (5.6 %), tannin (14.2-16.3 %), mucilage and wax (Umashankar *et al.,*1997).

Rhizomes of *B. ligulata* showed a presence of different chemical entities like;

Coumarins: bergenin, 11-0-galloyl bergenin, 11-O-P-hydroxy-benzoyl bergenin; 11-O-brotocatechuoyl bergenin, 4-0-galloyl bergenin;

Flavonoids: (+) afzelechin, avicularin, catechin, eriodictyol-7-O-β-D-glucopyranoside, reynoutrin; **Benzenoids:** arbutin, 6-O-P-hydroxy-benzoyl arbutin, 6-O-protocatechuoyl arbutin; 4-hydroxy benzoic acid;

Lactone: Idehcxan-5-olide, 3-(6'-O-P-hydroxy) (Chandrareddy *et al.,*1998; Fujii *et al.,*1996).

Compound name (Molecular Formula	Chemical Structure	Plant part	Reference No.
Afzelechin ($C_{15}H_{14}O_5$)		Rhizome	(Tucci *et al.*, 1969)
Leucocyanidin ($C_{15}H_{14}O_7$)		Rhizome	(Dixit *et al.*, 1989)
Bergenin ($C_{14}H_{16}O_9$)		Root, Rhizome	(Umashankar *et al.*, 1989)
Gallic acid ($C_7H_6O_5$)		Rhizome	(Dixit *et al.*, 1989)
Methyl gallate ($C_8H_8O_5$)		Rhizome	(Dixit *et al.*, 1989)

Tannic acid $(C_{76}H_{52}O_{46})$		Rhizome	(Dixit *et al.*,1989)
Catechin $(C_{15}H_{14}O_6)$		Rhizome	(Umashankar *et al.*,1997)
Sitoinoside I $(C_{51}H_{90}O_7)$		Rhizome	(Jain and Gupta ;1962) (Roy and Philip ;1981)
ß -Sitosterol $(C_{29}H_{50}O)$		Root	(Roy and Philip ;1981) (Umashankar *et al.*,1997)
ß -Sitosterol-D-Glucoside $(C_{35}H_{60}O_6)$		Root	(Roy and Philip ;1981) (Umashankar *et al.*,1997)

Glucose ($C_6H_{12}O_6$)		Rhizome	(Umashankar *et al.,*1997)
Avicularin ($C_{20}H_{18}O_{11}$)		Rhizome	(Fujii *et al.,*1996)
Eriodictyol-7-ß -D-glucopyranoside ($C_{21}H_{22}O_{11}$)		Rhizome	(Fujii *et al.,*1996)
Arbutin ($C_{12}H_{16}O_7$)		Rhizome	(Fujii *et al.,*1996)

Reynoutrin ($C_{20}H_{18}O_{11}$)		Rhizome	(Fujii *et al.*,1996) (Chandrareddy *et al.*,1998)
11-O-galloyl bergenin ($C_{21}H_{20}O_{13}$)		Rhizome	(Umashankar *et al.*,1997)
Pashaanolactone ($C_{19}H_{24}O_{10}$)		Rhizome	(Chandrareddy *et al.*,1998)
Catechin-7-O-ß -D-glucopyranoside ($C_{21}H_{24}O_{11}$)		Rhizome	(Umashankar *et al.*,1997)

Pharmacological activities

In view of the commercial, economic and medical importance of this crop, several workers have investigated the species pharmacognostically, chemically and also pharmacologically (Neelam & Krishnaswamy, 2001).

Medicinal Properties of Rhizome

Anti-inflammatory activity

Anti-inflammatory activity of aqueous extract of *Bergenia ciliata* rhizome performed and concluded that aqueous extract of *Bergenia ciliata* showed a potent and dose dependent anti-inflammatory effect comparable to Diclofenac sodium on induce paw edma in rats (Kumar *et al.,*2002).

Anti-tussive activity

The methanol extract of the rhizome of *Bergenia ciliata* Sternb. *(Saxifragaceae)* has been evaluated for its potential in a cough model induced by sulphur dioxide gas in mice. The extract exhibited significant antitussive activity in a dose-dependent manner, as compared with control. The antitussive activity of the extract was comparable to that of codeine phosphate (10 mg/kg body wt.), a standard anti-tussive agent. The extract at doses of 100, 200 and 300 mg/kg body wt. showed significant inhibition of cough reflex by 28.7, 33.9 and 44.2%, respectively, within 90 min of the experiment (Rajbhandari *et al.,*2007). The methanolic extract of *Bergenia ciliata* rhizome was screened for their antiviral activity against herpes simplex virus and influenza virus A by dye uptake assay. The methanolic extracts of *Bergenia ciliata* rhizome were found to be highly active against antiviral activity against HSV-1 (IC_{50} value 6.25µgml-1) and influenza virus A (IC_{50} values from 8 to 10 µgml-1) (Ruby *et al.,* 2012, Kakub *et al.,* 2007).

Antiulcer activity

Bergenia ciliata is used for the treatment of stomach disorders in the folk medicine of some areas of South East Asia. This study was designed to evaluate its gastroprotective effects on ethanol/HCl, indomethacin and pylorus ligation-induced gastric ulcers in rats. Doses of 15, 30 and 60 mg/kg between of the aqueous and methanol extracts of the rhizome were administered 1 h after ulcerogenic treatment. The animals were killed 3 h later, their stomachs removed and the mean area of ulcer lesion was determined. The weight of mucus and gastric acidity were also measured. The aqueous extract decreased the ulcer lesion ($p < 0.05$) in all models to a greater extent than the methanol extract, but at the higher doses the effect was reduced. In addition, the antiulcer activity appears to be mediated via cytoprotective effects conferred by enhancement of the mucosal barrier, rather than by prevention of gastric acid secretion or the lowering of pH and acidity (Ruby *et al.*, 2012, Stuffness *et al.*, 1990).

Anti-cancer activity

Methanolic and aqueous extract of *Bergenia ciliata* rhizome were found to have promising potential towards the development of drug that might be used to target tumours for chemoprevention/chemotherapy to check neoplastic growth and malignancy. Both extract showed concentration-dependent cytotoxicity in each of the three cell lines. According to the American national cancer institute, the IC_{50} value to consider a crude extract promising for development of anticancer drugs is lower than a limit threshold (30µg/ml).(Islam *et al.*,2002) IC_{50} value of both the extracts falls well within this prescribed threshold in all cell lines (except the aqueous extract with higher IC_{50} in help 3B cell lines) *B.ciliata* bear potent anti-neoplastic activities that may have prospective clinical use as precursor for preventive medicine (Bhandari *et al.*,2008).

Antioxidant activity

Methanolic and aqueous *B. ciliata* rhizome extracts were found to possess antioxidant activity, including reducing power, free radical scavenging activity and lipid peroxidation inhibition potential. The methanolic extract displayed greater potential in all antioxidant assays. It is interesting to note that the aqueous extract demonstrated considerably higher DNA protection, albeit lagging behind its methanolic counterpart as an antioxidant (Bhandari *et al.*, 2008).

Antidiabetic activity

50% aqueous –methanol extract of *Bergenia ciliata* rhizome lead to the isolation of two active compounds, (-)-3-O-galloylepicatechin and (-)-3-O-galloylcatechin.These isolated compounds demonstrated significant dose dependent enzyme inhibitory activities against rat intestinal α-glucosidase and porcine pancreatic α - amylase. IC50 value for sucrose, maltase and α-amylase were 560, 334 and 739 μM, respectively or [(-)-3-Ogalloylepicatechin] and 297, 150 and 401 μM, respectively for [(-)-3-O-galloylcatechin]. The anti-diabetic potential of *Pakhanbhed* could be helpful to develop medicinal preparations or nutraceutical and functional foods for diabetes and related symptoms (Venkatadri *et al.*, 2011).

Antiviral activity

In ethno-pharmacological screenings, plants used in Nepalese traditional medicine along with *B. ligulata* were evaluated for antiviral activity (Rajbhandari *et al.*, 2007).Methanolic and hydromethanolic extracts were assayed by *in-vitro* viral systems *viz.* influenza virus/MDCK cells and herpes simplex virus/vero cells and showed the highest antiinfluenza-viral activity with ID50 at 10 μg/ml (Rajbhandari *et al.*,2003, Tareq *et al.*,2005).

Anti-bradykinin activity

The alcoholic extract of *Bergenia ligulata* rhizome displays marked anti-bradykinin activity. Although, it does not affect the action of 5-HT and acetylcholine on isolated guinea pig ileum. It has been shown to potentiate the action of adrenaline on guinea-pig trachea and ileam muscle. Its cardiotoxic, antidiuretic and CNS depressant action on experimental models have been reported with large doses (WHO,1991). It is unlikely that these effects will be encountered with the doses in clinical use. In rats, the LD50 of the aqueous extract was 650 mg/kg intraperitoneally. It is widely used in the treatment of dysuria and renal failure, cystitis and crystalluria. Its anti-inflammatory property finds a use in the treatment of abscesses and cutaneous infections. It is also used in the treatment of dysentery and diarrhea (Garimella *et al.*, 2001).

Antibacterial activity

The antibacterial activity was tested using the disc diffusion method (Sajad *et al.*, 2010) measured by 10, 25 and 50 mg/ml plant extract. The zone of inhibition was calculated by measuring the minimum dimension of the zone of no microbial growth around the well. Aqueous, 50%ethanolic and methanolic extracts of *B. ligulata* rhizomes were tested for their ability to inhibit the growth of *E. coli*, *B. subtilis*, and *S. aureus* at the dose levels of 10, 25 or 50 mg/ml for each extract. At a dose level of 50 mg/ml, the antibacterial effect was most significant. Incidentally, the antibacterial effect of the extracts at this level was comparable to ciprofloxacin (25 mg/ml). The results clearly suggest that *B. ligulata* possesses a strong antibacterial activity (Winter *et al.*, 1962).

Antiurolithic activity

The traditional use of *B. ligulata* for kidney disorders is also supported by the experimental studies (Basant *et al.*, 2008, Gurocak *et al.*, 2006, Sharma *et al.*, 2001). The methanolic extract of rhizomes of *B. ligulata* and the isolated constituents like bergenin were compared for urolithiatic activity in albino rats. *B. ligulata* rhizomes inhibited CaC_2O_4 crystal formation as well as crystal aggregation and exhibited antioxidant effect against 1, 1-diphenyl-2-picrylhydrazyl free radical and lipid peroxidation in *in-vitro* conditions. In a modified animal model (male wistar rats) of urolithiasis which developed by addition of 0.75% ethylene glycol in drinking water, methanolic extract (5–10 mg/kg) of *B. ligulata* rhizomes prevented CaC_2O_4 crystal deposition in the renal tubules. Polyuria, weight loss, impairment of renal function and oxidative stress, due to the lithogenic treatment were also prevented by *B. ligulata* extract. Unlike the untreated animals, ethylene glycol intake did not cause excessive hyperoxaluria and hypocalciuria in *B. ligulata* treated groups and there was a significant increase in the urinary Mg2+. These data indicated the antiurolithic activity of *B. ligulata* mediated possibly through CaC_2O_4 crystal inhibition, diuretic, hypermagneseuric and antioxidant effects which rationalizes its medicinal use in urolithiasis (Bashir *et al.*,2009). Methanolic extract of *B. ligulata* and bergenin exhibited marked dissolution of urinary calculi both in kidney and urine constituents (Satish and Umashankar,2006). *In-vitro* antilithiatic / anticalcification activities of various extracts of *B. ligulata* and *Dolichos biflorus* individually and in combination were tested by the homogeneous precipitation method. The extracts were compared with an aqueous extract of 'Cystone' (Formulation of Himalaya Company, India) for their activities. Extracts of *D. biflorus* showed activity almost equivalent to 'Cystone' while *B. ligulata* showed less activity and the combination was not as active as the individual extracts. After this study, it was concluded that the active constituent/s seem to be non-protein, non-tannin molecule/s which may act through inhibition of calcium and phosphate accumulation (Garimella *et al.*, 2001). Low doses of *B. ligulata* extract (0.5 mg/kg of alcoholic extract) promote diuresis in rats, but higher doses of 100 mg/kg reduce the urine output and the diuresis produced by urea (Panda, 2002). In comparative study, the aqueous extracts of *B. ligulata* produced maximum inhibition of the growth of Calcium oxalate monohydrate (COM) crystals than *Tribulus terrestris* (Joshi *et al.*,2005). From this study it was hypothesized that the biomacromolecules from *B.*

ligulata seem to play an important role in the inhibition of COM crystals.

Analgesic activity

The analgesic activity was evaluated by using hydroalcoholic extract of rhizomes of *B. ligulata*, (250 mg/kg) administering intra-gastrically in the mouse by employing hot plate and tail clip methods (Abraham *et al.*, 1986) Consequently it was inferred that the extract was devoid of analgesic activity.

Medicinal activity of root
Hepatoprotective activity

The ethanolic extracts of root of *Bergenia ligulata* were assessed for hepatoprotective activity in albino rats that was compared with standard drugs. Acute toxicity studies were carried out for ethanolic extract of *Bergenia ligulata* root on healthy Swiss albino mice of body weight 25- 35g by using Up and Down or Stair case method (Rai *et al.*, 1997). Evaluation of the hepatoprotective activity was done by measuring the levels of serum glutamate pyruvate transaminase (SGPT), serum glutamate oxaloacetate transminase (SGOT) serum alkaline phosphatase and total bilirubin levels (Shukla *et al.*, 1996). The ethanolic extract of the roots of *Bergenia ligulata* was found to produce significant activity (Anonymous , 2006).

Diuretic activity

The ethanolic extracts of root of *Bergenia ligulata* were assessed for diuretic activity in albino rats that was compared with standard drugs. For evaluation of the diuretic activity Lipschits method, was used (Kuppast and Nayak,2005;Murugesan *et al.*,2005;Joshi *et al.*,2005).It was done by measuring the volume of urine collected at the end of 5 hrs and Na+,K+ and Cl- concentration in urine. The ethanolic extract of the roots of *Bergenia ligulata* was found to produce significant activity (Anonymous, 2006).The extracts of

Bergenia ligulata root were studied in the presence of artificial reference urine (ARU) and human urine (HU) the growth behaviours of CHPD crystals grew within the rings. The addition of aqueous extract of *B. ligulata* to the calcium chloride in the supernatant solution modified the diffusion process and hence the periodic precipitation and the number of liesegang rings.The maximum length of the crystals was reduced due to inhibition produced by the addition of aqueous extract of *B.ligulata* the HU aqueous extract (AE) of *B. ligulata* contained a large number of salts and organic molecule. And their complex formation may have promoted the effect on growth of CHPD crystals .But when they are added separately to $CaCl_2$ they inhibit the growth of crystals. This suggests that these solutions separately inhibit the growth of crystals in in–vitro condition. But mixing with HU (humane urine), it changes their behavior markedly. The diuretic nature of AE/*B.ligulata* seems to be important in the remedy rather than their inhibitive nature (Arora *et al.*, 2011).

Medicinal activity of combined plant part (root, rhizome and leaves)

Antipyretic activity

The ethanolic (95%) extracted of roots, rhizomes and leaves and aqueous extract of whole plant of *Bergenia ligulata* Wall in yeast induced fever in albino rats of wistar strain were assessed for antipyretic activity (Naik *et al.*, 1972).The yield of semisolid mass (w/w) was obtained as ethanol extract of roots (13.36%), ethanol extract of rhizomes (15.12%), ethanol extract of leaves (11.02%) and aqueous extract of whole plant (09.21%). Acute toxicity studies were carried out for all the extracts of *Bergenia ligulata Wall* on healthy swiss albino mice of body weight 25-35g by using Up and Down or Stair case method (Shukla *et al.*, 1996). The suspension of all the extracts of *Bergenia ligulata* Wall was prepared in 5% gum acacia and employed for assessment of antipyretic activity at the dose of

(300 and 500mg/kgbody weight)(Mitra *et al.*, 2010). The standard drug used was paracetamol (200mg/kg.p.o) (Naik *et al.*, 1972). Rectal temperature of experimental animals was recorded at a time interval of 1hr, 2hr, 3hr, 4hr and 5 hr after drug administration for evaluation of antipyretic activity. The ethanolic extract of roots and rhizomes of *Bergenia ligulata* Wall at a dose of 500mg/kg.p.o decreased the yeast induced fever in experimental animals (Singh *et al.*, 2009) The ethanolic extracts of root of *Bergenia ligulata* were assessed for antipyretic activities in albino rats that were compared with standard drug. The assessment of Antipyretic activity was carried out using Brewer's Yeast induced pyrexia method in wistar rats(Pelczar *et al.*, 1993). Rectal temperature was recorded at a time interval of 0, 30 min, 1 hr, 2 hr and 3 hr after drug administration for evaluation of antipyretic activity the ethanolic extract of the roots of *Bergenia ligulata* was found to produce significant antipyretic activity (Anonymous , 2006).

Germplasm status

At present, over 30 species were found in the globe and all of them have high pharmaceutical values, in addition, it can also be used in horticulture, food and cosmetic. But now, wild species of *Bergenia* possessing high application values have gradually been becoming lacking, nearly to the brink of extinction, because of destruction of ecological environment and excessive excavation. *Bergenia* is mainly distributed in Asia, involved in East Asia, the south-eastern regions of Central Asia and northern regions of South Asia (Chandra Reddy *et al.*, 1998; Zhou *et al.*, 2007). According to The International Plant Names Index (www.ipni.org), there are 32 species in the world (Table 1).

No.	Species ID code	Full name
32 *Berginia* species in the world		
1	*Bergenia* 331394-2	*Bergenia* Moench
	36961-1	*Bergenia* Moench
	Boriss.) J.T.Pan926908-1	*Bergenia* sect. *Ciliatae* (
	J.T.Pan 926010-1	*Bergenia* sect. *Scopulosae*
2	*Bergenia beesiana* C.Schneider790352-1	*Bergenia beesiana* Hort. ex
3	*Bergenia biflora* Moench 790353-1	*Bergenia biflora*
	790354-1	*Bergenia bifolia* Moench
4	*Bergenia ciliata* Engl. 790357-1	*Bergenia ciliata* A.Braun ex
	790355-1	*Bergenia ciliata* Stein
	Sternb. 790356-1	*Bergenia ciliata* (Haw.)
5	*Bergenia cordifolia* 790358-1	*Bergenia cordifolia* Sternb.
6	*Bergenia coreana* 790359-1	*Bergenia coreana* Nakai
		Bergenia coreana Nakai

790360-1

7	*Bergenia crassifolia*
Bergenia crassifolia (L.) Fritsch var. *sajanensis* Stepanov 77099297-1
Bergenia crassifolia (L.) Fritsch 790361-1

8	*Bergenia delavayi* *Bergenia delavayi* Engl. 790362-1

9	*Bergenia emeiensis*
Bergenia emeiensis C.Y.Wu ex J.T.Pan 934834-1
Bergenia emeiensis C.Y.Wu ex J.T.Pan var. *rubellina* J.T.Pan 981392-1

10	*Bergenia fortunei* *Bergenia fortunei* Stein 790363-1

11	*Bergenia gorbunovii*
Bergenia gorbunovii B.Fedtsch. & Boriss. 790365-1
Bergenia gorbunovii B.Fedtsch.   790364-1

12	*Bergenia himalaica* *Bergenia himalaica* Boriss. 790366-1

13	*Bergenia hissarica* *Bergenia hissarica* Boriss. 790367-1

14	*Bergenia ligulata* *Bergenia ligulata* (Wall.) Engl. 790368-1
Bergenia ligulata (Wall.) Engl. 790369-1

43

15	*Bergenia media* 790370-1	*Bergenia media* Engl.
16	*Bergenia milesii* 790371-1	*Bergenia milesii* Stein
17	*Bergenia × newryensis* 790372-1	*Bergenia × newryensis* Yeo
18	*Bergenia orbicularis* 790373-1	*Bergenia orbicularis* Stein
19	*Bergenia ornata* 790375-1 790374-1	*Bergenia ornata* Stein & Guillaumin *Bergenia ornata* Stein
20	*Bergenia pacifica* 790376-1	*Bergenia pacifica* Komarov
21	*Bergenia pacumbis* Ham. ex D.Don) C.Y.Wu & J.T.Pan 945348-1	*Bergenia pacumbis* (Buch.-
22	*Bergenia purpurascens* *purpurascens* Engl. 790377-1	*Bergenia*
	Bergenia purpurascens (Hook.f. & Thomson) Engl. 790378-1	
	Bergenia purpurascens (Hook.f. & Thomson) Engl. var. *Sessilis* H.Chuang 1020959-1	
23	*Bergenia schmidtii*	*Bergenia schmidtii* (Regel)

Silva Tarouca790379-1	
24 *Bergenia × schmidtii* *Bergenia × schmidtii* (Regel) Silva Tarouca , prospec. & Yeo 790380-1	
25 *Bergenia scopulosa* *Bergenia scopulosa* T.P.Wang 790381-1	
26 *Bergenia smithii* *Bergenia smithii* Engl. 790382-1	
27 *Bergenia spathulata* *Bergenia spathulata* Nagels ex Guillaumin 790383-1	
28 *Bergenia stracheyi* *Bergenia stracheyi* Stein 790384-1 *Bergenia stracheyi* (Hook.f. & Thomson) Engl. 790385-1	
29 *Bergenia thysanodes* *Bergenia thysanodes* (Lindl.) C.Schneider 790386-1	
30 *Bergenia tianquanensis* *Bergenia* *tianquanensis* J.T.Pan 981391-1	
31 *Bergenia ugamica* *Bergenia ugamica* V.N.Pavlov 790387-1	
32 *Bergenia yunnanensis* *Bergenia yunnanensis* Hort. 790388-1	

*Same species could probably be found by different researchers in different regions, so some species have several full names, but one full name only has unique ID code
. (Source : www.ipni.org)

Need for Conservation

Being a high potential medicinal plant it has been depleting from their natural habitat. This depletion is due to high pressure for their over exploitation through shifting cultivation, expansion of urbanization, agricultural land and road development as well as some natural calamities like land sliding, protection from wild animals and unwanted forest practices like fire, and soil degradation etc.Acute pressure exerted over Berginia through unscientific collection of drugs from natural habitat only has made a need for utmost necessary for conservation. Many studies have confirmed that pharmaceutical companies are also responsible for inefficient, imperfect, informal, and opportunistic marketing of medicinal plants. (Kala, 2003)

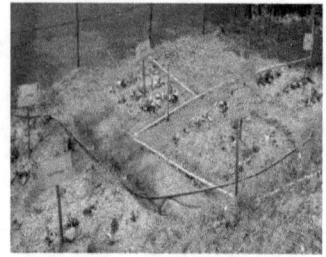 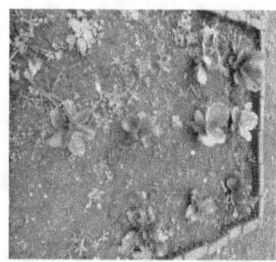

Fig 3. Field view of different germplasm of Pakhanbhed

Realizing the importance, it has been felt necessary to undertake both *in-situ,* as well as *ex-situ* conservation. Although species conservation is achieved most effectively through the management of wild populations and natural habitats i.e. *in situ* conservation (Ramsay et. al.,2006, Fay,1992, Negash *et al.,*2001). *Ex-situ* conservation may be done in the form of depositing the live materials in the gene bank, establishing field gene bank and also promoting cultivation of medicinal plants (Hussain and Hore,2006) and also maintaining plants through long-term preservation of plant Propagules in plant tissue culture repositories (Bennun *et al.,*2010). These *Ex-situ* techniques can be used to complement *in situ* methods and, in some instances, may be the only option for some species ((Ramsay *et.al,* 2006, Fay, 1992, Negash *et al.,* 2001).

Challenges to commercial cultivation of Berginia

The best way to ensure the continuous supply of best quality and uniform herbal product of Berginia can be obtained by domestication, through adopting correct agro-techniques to produce quality raw material. However, n-number of lacking, creating a huge gap to popularizing Pakhanbhed cultivation. These are as follows:

1. Good Agricultural Practices (**GAP**) and Good Agricultural Collection Practices (**GACP**) for Berginia not yet developed.

2. **Standardize agro-technology** yet to be worked out for region and altitude specific for cultivation of Berginia.

3. **Capacity to outcompete native species**

   Extensive survey should be carried out to identify best superior clone which can compete the foreign one in all the parameters. During the survey genetic diversity and variations needs to be observed to find out best clone. Exact harvesting time in relation to berginin content needs to be standardized as secondary metabolites are main interest compound. Promising clone can be multiplied and distributed to the local growers for planting.

4. Variety for Berginia is not yet developed for cultivation.

Genetic improvement is aimed at improving the yield and quality of Berginia for making it suitable for cultivation and to provide higher economic return. Selection of desirable and superior genotypes is the key of all applied genetic improvement programmes. The objective is to obtain sufficient amount of genetic gain as quickly and inexpensively as possible. All the methods of selection are based on general principle of choosing most desirable individuals for use as parents in breeding and production programmes. The literature on this species is scanty and no scientific study had been made so far on intra-specific variations, genetic improvement, developing cultivars and cultivation practice etc.

5. Overconsumption makes it vulnerable to local extinction.

Berginia grows luxuriantly in all the North Eastern States. Due to unscientific harvesting and over exploitation such unlimited plant bio-resources or natural genetic stock, that could be converted into immediate cash and be used in sustainable manners, is going to be extinct.

6. Depletion of gene pool of Berginia.

The natural gene pool of Berginia is depleting rapidly mainly due to biotic pressure and developmental activities. The major causes are seedling mortality due to browsing and grazing, depletion of natural seed bank and conversion of forest lands for cultivation and construction purposes etc. To conserve the depleting gene pool of the different species, field gene banks needs to be established at different places region-wise, altitude-wise for enriching the genetic diversity in field gene bank. Demonstration farm needs to be established for creating awareness through demonstration and training programmes for the local people.

Conclusion

The pakhanbhed can play vital role for improving the rural livelihood in hills track of north-eastern India. It has potential use in herbal medicine. Due to biotic pressure and developmental activities are leading to depletion of its genetic resources in natural stock. Superior genotype, intra- specific variation, genetic improvement, development of region-specific cultivars, Good agricultural practice, Agro-economic needs to be worked out for popularizing cultivation of Berginia. Domestication of the species can contribute to economic growth and improve needs of the communities. This will in turn help in conserving the species diversity and gene pool of the species. Proper post harvest management with processing and value addition facilities needs to be standardized for enhancing the economic growth of pakhanbhed growers. Cultivation of Berginia can be done in waste lands which remain barren/fellow/wall in the hill track for multipurpose use. Hand on Training on cultivation, management practices, proper harvesting, drying and storage can be conducted for creating awareness among the farming community. Training on preparation of herbal product and packaging can be conducted for encouraging the rural entrepreneurship.

REFERENCES

Abraham, Z. Bhakuni, S.D., Garg H.S., Goel, A.K., Mehrotra, B.N, Pathak, G.K. (1986). "Screening of Indian Medicinal Plants for biological activity: Part XII". *Indian Journal of Experimental Biology*. 24:48-68.

Anonymous (1988). "The Wealth of India: A Dictionary of Indian Raw Materials & Industrial Products". New Delhi, India: CSIR Publications;:119-120.

Anonymous (1989). Royal Horticultural Society." Ground Cover Plants". Cassells. ISBN 0-304-31089-1 A handy little booklet from the R.H.S.

Anonymous (1991).WHO, in Progress Report by the Director General, Document NO.A44/20, 22 March, World health organization. Geneva.

Anonymous (1998 and 2001). "Progress Report of the Project .Studies on Medicinal Plants of Sikkim". State Council of Science and Technology for Sikkim.

Anonymous (2002)."Indian Herbal Pharmacopoeia". Revised edition. Mumbai: IDMA Publication;79-87.

Anonymous (2006) "A Manual on Participatory Inventory and Management of Pakhenbed (*Bergenia ciliata syn. Bergenia ligulata*)", Based on results of case studies from six CFs of Ramechhap District. Nepal Swiss Community Forestry Project (NSCFP) Date: April 07, 2006 Ref. No.24/062/63.

Anonymous (2009). "Guide to Growing Bergenia Plants". The Garden Helper. Retrieved 09-06-2016.

Anonymous (2009). The Ayurvedic Pharmacopoeia of India part- I volume – I

Anupama. (2014). "Pashanbheda: A great herb to dissolve kidney stone and more."*Bimbima*.21October2014,http://www.bimbima.com/health/post/2014/10/21/pashanbhedabergenia-ligulata.aspx

Arora, R., Chawla, R., Marwah, R., Arora, P., Sharma, R.K., Kaushi,V., Goel, R., Kaur, A., Silambarasan, M., Tripathi, R.P. and Bhardwaj, J.R. (2011). " Potential of complementary alternative medicine in preventive management of novel H1N1 Flu (Swine Flu) Pandemic: Thwarting potential disasters in the bud". *Evidence-Based Complementary and Alternative Medicine.* 11-16

Basant, B., Chaurasia, O.P., Zakwan, A. and Singh, S.B.(2008). "Traditional medicinal plants of cold desert, Ladakh-used against kidney and urinary disorders". *Journal of Ethnopharmacology.* 118:331-339.

Bashir, S. and Gilani, A. (2009). "Antiurolithic effect of *Bergenia ligulata* rhizome: An explanation of the underlying mechanisms". *Journal of Ethnopharmacology*.122:106-116.

Bhandari, M.R., Anurakkun, N.J., Gao, H. and Kawabata, J.(2008). "α - Glucosidase and α –amylase inhibitory activities of Nepalese medicinal herb Pakhanbhed (*Bergenia ciliata*, Haw.)" *Food Chemistry*. 106:; 247–252.

Bhāvaprakāsha: Bhāvaprakāsha Nighantu. Published by Chaukhamba Sanskrit Series officeBanaras. Haritkyādi Vargah: 103)

Brickell,C. (1990). "The RHS Gardener's Encyclopedia of Plants and Flowers," Dorling Kindersley Publishers Ltd. ISBN 0-86318-386-7

Kala, C. P. (2003). "Commercial exploitation and conservation status of high value medicinal plants across the borderline of India and Nepal in Pithoragarh," *Indian Forester*. vol. 129, pp. 80–84.

Chandra Reddy, U.D., Chawla, A.S., Mundkinajeddu, D., Maurya, R. and Handa, S.S. (1998). "Paashaanolactone from *Bergenia ligulata*". *Phytochemistry,* 47: 907-909.

Chauhan, R., Ruby, K.M. and Dwived, J. (2012). " Pashanbheda a Golden Herb of Himalaya: A Review". *Int. J. Pharm. Sci. Rev. Res.* 15(2), 2012; no 05, 24-30

Dixit, B.S., Srivastava, S.N. (1989). "Tannin constituents of *Bergenia ligulata* roots". *Indian Journal of Natural Products*.5:24-25.

Dorling, Kindersley (2008). "RHS A-Z encyclopedia of garden plants". United Kingdom: p. 1136. ISBN 1405332964.

Fay, M. F. (1992). "Conservation of rare and endangered plants using *in vitro* methods," *In Vitro Cellular & Developmental Biology— Plant*, vol. 28, pp. 1–4,.

Fujii, M., Miyaichi, Y. and Tomimori, T. (1996). " Studies on Nepalese crude drugs on the phenolic constituents of the rhizomes of *Bergenia ciliata* (Haw.)" Sternb. *Natural Medicine*.50:404-7.

Fujii, M., Miyaichi, Y. And Tomimori, T. (1996). "Studies on Nepalese crude drugs on the phenolic constituents of the rhizomes of *Bergenia ciliata* (Haw.) Sternb". *Natural Medicine*.50:404-7.

Garimella, T.S., Jolly, C.I. and Narayanan,S. (2001). "In vitro study on antilithiatic activity of seeds of *Dolichos biflorus* and rhizome of *Begenia ligulata wall." Phytother: res.,* 15(4):;351-356.

Govindchari, T. (1992). " Selected Medicinal Plants of India". Bombay: Tata Press Ltd; p. 53-54.

Grierson A.J.C. and Long, D.G. (1987). "Flora of Bhutan" (Vol. 1, Part 3). Royal Botanic Garden, Edinburgh.;492.

Gurocak, S. and Kupeli, B.(2006) "Consumption of historical and current phytotherapeutic agents for urolithiasis: A Critical Review". *The Journal of Urology*.176:450-455.

Hafidh, R.R., Abdulamir, A.S., Jahanshiri, F., Abas, F., AbuBakar, F. and Sekawi, Z.(2009). "Asia is the mine of natural antiviral products for public health", *The Open Complementary Med.J.*58-68.

Huxley, A.(1992). "The New RHS Dictionary of Gardening." MacMillan Press ISBN 0-333-47494-5 .

Islam, M., Azhar, I., Azhar, F., Usmanghani, K., Gill, M.A., Ahmad, A. and Shahabuddin. (2002). "Evalution of antibacterial activity of *Bergenia ciliata*". *A Pakistan J Pharmaceutical Sci.* 15(2);21-27.

Jain MK, Gupta RJ (1962) " Isolation of bergenin from *Saxifraga ligulata* Wall". *Indian Chemical Society.*39:559-560.

Jain, M.K. and Gupta, R.J. (1962). "Isolation of bergenin from *Saxifraga ligulata* Wall". *Indian Chemical Society.* 39:559-560.

Joshi, V.S., Parekh, B.B., Joshi, M.J. and Ashok Vaidya, D.B. (2005). " Inhibition of the growth of urinary calcium hydrogen phosphate dihydrate crystals with aqueous extracts of *Tribulus terrestris* and *Bergenia ligulata*". *Urol Res* . 33; 80–86.

Joshi, V.S., Parekh, B.B., Joshi, M.J. and Vaidya, A.D. (2005). " Inhibition of the growth of urinary calcium hydrogen phosphate dihydrate crystals with aqueous extracts of *Tribulus terrestris* and *Bergenia ligulata*". *Urological Research.*33:80.

Kakub, G. and Gulfraz, M. (2007). "Cytoprotective effects of *Bergenia ciliata Sternb,* extract on gastric ulcer in rats". *Phytother Res.*21(12);1217-20.

Kirtikar, K. and Basu, B. (2005). "Textbook of Indian Medicinal Plants". Volume II, 2nd ed. Dehradun, India: International Book Distributors; 993-994. .

Kumar, V. and Shah, G. (2002). " Anti-inflammatory activity of aqueous extract of *Bergenia ciliata".Journal Of Natural Remedies.* 2; 189-190.

Kuppast, I.J. and Nayak, P.V.(2005) "Diuretic activity of *Cordial dichotoma* forster fruits". *Ind. J Pharm.Edu. Res.* 39(4);67-74.

Rands,M. R.W., Adams, W. M. and Bennun, L. (2010). "Biodiversity conservation: challenges beyond," *Science*, vol. 329, no.5997, pp. 1298–1303,.

Manjunatha, S.N. (2010). " Pharmacognostic finger print profile of a controversial drug Paashanabheda". M. Pharm Dissertation, Rajiv Gandhi University of Health Sciences, Karnataka, India.

Mehra, P.N. and Raina, M.K. (1971). "Pharmacognosy of Pashaanbheda". *Indian Journal of Pharmacology.*33:126.

Mitra, S.K., Saxena, E. And Babu, U.V. (2010). " Herbal composition for maintaining/caring the skin around the eye, methods of preparing the same and uses", US patent 7;785,637

Murugesan, T., Manikandan, L. and Suresh, K.B. (2000). "Evalution of diuretic potential of *Jussiaea suffruticosa linn.* extract in rats". *Ind.J.Pharm.Sci.* 150-153.

Naik, S.R., Kalyanpur, S.N. and Sheth, U.K. (1972). "Effect of anti-inflammatory drugs on glutithione levels and liver succinic dehydrogenase activity in carrageenan edema and cotton pellet granuloma in rat". *Biochemical Pharmacology.* 21;511-516.

Negash, A., Krens,F., Schaart,J. and Visser,B. (2001). "*In vitro* conservation of enset under slow-growth conditions," *Plant Cell, Tissue and Organ Culture*, vol. 66, no. 2, pp. 107–111.

Panda, H.(2002). "Herbs Cultivation & Medicinal Uses", National Institute of Industrial Research, New Delhi. :220-222.

Pelczar, M.J., Chan, E.C.S. and Krieg, N.R.(1993). "Microbiology". 5thed. MC Graw Hill.; 578.

Phillips, R. and Rix, M. (1991)."Perennials Volumes 1 and 2". Pan Books ISBN 0-330-30936-9

Rai, R.P., Rajendra Babu M. and Rao, K.R.V. (1997). "Studies on antipyretic, analgesic and hypoglycaemic activities of root of *Gynandropsis gynandra linn.*" *Indian Drugs*.34(12); 690-693.

Rajbhandari, M., Mentel, R, Jha PK, Chaudhary, R.P., Bhattarai, S., Gewali, M.B., Karmacharya, N., Hipper, M. and Lindequist, U. (2007). "Antiviral Activity of Some Plants Used in Nepalese Traditional Medicine". *eCAM*. 6(4);517–522.

Rajbhandari, M., Wegner, U., Julich, M., Schopke, T. and Mentel, R. (2001). "Screening of Nepalese medicinal plants for antiviral activity". *Journal of Ethnopharmacology*.74:251-255.

Rajbhandari, M., Wegner, U., Schopke, T., Lindequist, U., Mentel, R. (2003). "Inhibitory effect of *Bergenia ligulata* on influenza virus" . *Die Pharmazie;*58:268-271.

Rice. G. (1988). " Growing from Seed". *Volume 2.* Thompson and Morgan.

Very readable magazine with lots of information on propagation. An interesting article on Ensete ventricosum.

Roy, D.H.and Philip, J.H.(1981). "Phenolic constituents of the cell walls of Dicotyledons". *Biochemical Systematics and Ecology*.9:189-203.

Ruby, K., Chauhan, R., Sharma, S. and Dwivedi, J. (2012). " Polypharmacological activities of Bergenia species". *International Journal of Pharmaceutical Sciences Review and Research.* 13(1); 100-110

Sajad, T., Zargar, A., Ahmad, T., Bader, G.N., Naime, M. and Ali, S. (2010). "Antibacterial and Anti-inflammatory Potential *Bergenia ligulata"*. *Am. J. Biomed. Sci.* 2(4);313-321.

Satish, H. and Umashankar, D. (2006). " Comparative study of methanolic extract of *Bergenia ligulata* Yeo. with isolated constituent bergenin in urolithiatic rats". *Biomed.*1:80-87.

Sharma, H.K., Chhangte, L. and Dolui, A.K. (2001). " Traditional medicinal plants in Mizoram, India". *Fitoterapia*.72:146-161.

Shukla, D.S., Ravishankar,V.J. and Bhavasar, B. (1996). "Preliminary study on the hepatoprotective activity of methanolic extract of *Paederia foetida* leaf". *Fitoterapia* . LX VII (2); 106-109.

Singh, A and Sandhu, A. (2005). "A Dictionary of Medicinal Plants". New Delhi: Sundeep Publishers; p. 46

Singh, N., Juyal,V., Gupta, A.K. and Gahlot, M. (2009). "Evaluation of ethanolic extract of root of *Bergenia ligulata* for hepatoprotective, diuretic and antipyretic activites". *J Pharmacy Research.* 2(5);958-960.

Srivastava, S. and Rawat, A. (2008). "Botanical and phytochemical comparison of three *Bergenia* species". *Journal of Scientific and Industrial Research*.67:65-72.

Stuffness, M and Pezzuto, J.M.(1990). "Assay related to cancer drug discovery". In Hostettmann K.(ed). Methods in plant biochemistry. Assays for Bioactivity, 6. Academic press.London.;71-133.

Tareq, M., Khan, H., Ather, A., Thompson, K. and Gambari, R. (2005)."Extracts and molecules from medicinal plants against herpes simplex viruses". *Antiviral Research*; 67:107-119.

Thomas. G. S. (1990). *"Plants for Ground Cover"* J. M. Dent & Sons ; ISBN 0-460-12609-1 An excellent detailled book on the subject, very comprehensive.

Tucci, P.A., Delle, M.F. and Marini-Beholo, B.G. (1969). " Occurrence of (+)- afzelchin in *Saxifraga ligulata"*. *Ann First Super Sanita.*5:555-556.

Tucci, P.A., Delle, M.F. and Marini-Beholo, B.G. (1969). "Occurrence of (+)- afzelchin in *Saxifraga ligulata."* *Ann First Super Sanita.*5:555-556.

Udupa, K.N., Chaturvedi, G.N. and Tripathi, S.N.(1970). "Advances in Research in Indian Medicine", Banaras Hindu University: Varanasi;:77.

Umashankar, D., Chawla, A., Deepak, M., Singh, D. and Handa S(1999). " High pressure liquid chromatographic determination of bergenin and (+)- afzelechin from different parts of Paashaanbheda (*Bergenia ligulata*)". *Phytochemical Analysis.*10:44.

Umashankar, D.C. (1997). " Phytochemical and anti-inflammatory investigations of *Bergenia ligulata".* Ph.D. thesis, Punjab University, Chandigarh,

Sarasan, V. Cripps, R. and Ramsay, M. M. (2006). "Conservation *in vitro* of threatened plants-progress in the past decade," *In Vitro Cellular and Developmental Biology—Plant,* vol. 42, no. 3, pp 206–214.

Venkatadri, R., Guha G. and Rangasamy, A.K. (2011). "Anti-neoplastic activity of *Bergenia ciliata* rhizome". *J Pharmacy Res.* 4(2);443-445.

Winter, C.A., Ristey, E.A. and Nuss, G.W. (1962). " Carrageenan induced edema in hind paw of the rat as an assay for antiinflammatory drugs". Proceeding of Society of *Experimental Biology Medicine* 111;544-552.

Zhou, G.Y., Li, W.C. and Guo, F.G. (2007). "Resource investigation and observation of biological characteristics of *Bergenia purpurascens* (Hook. f. et Thoms.) Engl." *Chin. Agric. Sci. Bull.,* 23: 390-392.